BLUEPRINTS
Computer-Based Case
Simulation Review
USMLE Step 3

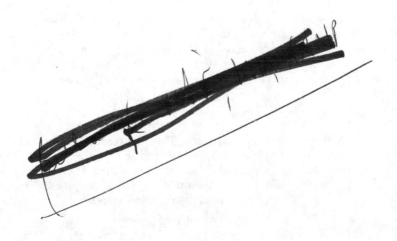

Praise for
Blueprints Computer-Based Case Simulation Review
USMLE Step 3

"I did not realize the need for help in the case-based portion of Step 3 until I read this. I just figured I'd learn enough during internship to go through it easily, but the hints/tricks are very helpful."

—Intern, Transitional Year

"I think a guide for this portion of the exam is very useful. In general, I think most students feel it is the 'easier' part of the test. But it is not intuitive and there are definitely a few pointers that help in figuring out strategy. Just playing with the case examples does not address some of these lessons that can help a student optimize their score."

—Clinical and Research Fellow, Department of Dermatology

"I think that this book is a wonderful idea! The CCS portion of Step 3 exam is so clunky [and] clumsy. I never did quite get it, or understand what the heck I was supposed to be doing. While the portion of the exam was fun in theory, there were many problems in learning the 'rules' of interface. Also, the relatively few number of cases that were available on the practice CD did not give me enough time to get familiar with the program."

—Clinical Fellow, Psychiatry, PGY-IV Chief Resident

"This would be a great book for residents to purchase. Not many books provide specific advice for the CCS like this one does. This is must-have. The sample cases are very stereotypical of what to expect on Step 3—I had some very similar if not the same type of cases. I just finished step 3 today, and I wish I would have had this book to [prepare]!"

—PGY-1, Family Practice Resident

"I think the sample cases are great. They are accurate in terms of content and types of scenarios. I appreciated the curves thrown in with the secondary diagnoses and the attention to setting. These are accurate to the exam, and the items that are difficult to pick up on in computer-based simulation vs. reality."

—General Surgery Resident

BLUEPRINTS
Computer-Based Case Simulation Review USMLE Step 3

Carter E. Wahl, MD
Resident in Pathology
University of California, San Diego
San Diego, California

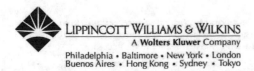

LIPPINCOTT WILLIAMS & WILKINS
A **Wolters Kluwer** Company

Philadelphia • Baltimore • New York • London
Buenos Aires • Hong Kong • Sydney • Tokyo

351 West Camden Street
Baltimore, Maryland 21201-2436 USA

530 Walnut Street
Philadelphia, Pennsylvania 19106-3621 USA

Printed in the United States of America

Library of Congress Cataloging-in-Publication Data

Wahl, Carter E.
  Blueprints computer-based case simulation review : USMLE step 3 / Carter E. Wahl.
    p. ; cm.
  Includes bibliographical references and index.
  ISBN-13: 978-1-4051-0445-6 (pbk.)
  ISBN-10: 1-4051-0445-7 (pbk.)
  1. Clinical medicine—Case studies—Computer simulation. 2. Physicians—
Licenses—United States—Examinations—Study guides.
  [DNLM: 1. Clinical Medicine—methods—Case Reports. 2. Clinical Medicine—
methods—Examination Questions. 3. Computer Simulation. WB 18.2 W136b 2005]
  I. Title: Computer-based case simulation review. II. Title.

  RC66.W24 2005
  616'.0076—dc22

                                                                        2004005967

Editor: Donna Balado
Managing Editor: Kathleen Scogna
Marketing Manager: Emilie Linkins

To purchase additional copies of this book call our customer service department at **(800) 638-3030** or fax orders to **(301) 824-7390**. International customers should call **(301) 714-2324**.

Visit **Lippincott Williams & Wilkins on the Internet: http://www.lww.com**. Lippincott Williams & Wilkins customer service representatives are available from 8:30 am to 6:00 pm, EST, Monday through Friday, for telephone access.

                                                                              07
                                                              5 6 7 8 9 10

For Eric J. and Elizabeth M. Wahl

Contents

Reviewers . . . .*ix*

Preface . . . .*xi*

1 Scheduling and Preparing for the Exam 1
Pre-Exam Requirements
Exam Preparation
Advice for International Medical Graduates

2 Conquering the CCS 5
Initial Management Stage
Watching and Waiting

3 Managing Time 14
Advancing the Clock
Completing a Case

4 CCS versus Reality 18
How Realistic is the CCS?
General Tips on Ordering

5 Scoring 22
Multiple-Choice Scoring
CCS Scoring

6 Sample Cases 26
Predicting Your Case Topics
Sample Cases

Appendix *73*

References *75*

Index *76*

Reviewers

Bhushan S. Agharkar, MD
Chief Resident, Psychiatry
Emory University Hospitals
Emory University School of Medicine
Atlanta, Georgia

Brooke Buckley, MD
General Surgery Resident
Fairview Hospital
Cleveland, Ohio

Jacquelⁱne Dolev, MD
Department of Dermatology
University of California, San Francisco
San Francisco, California

Amy Gull, DO
Intern, Transitional Year
Eastmoreland Hospital
Portland, Oregon

Matthew F. Kalady, MD
Senior Resident, General Surgery
Duke University Medical Center
Duke University School of Medicine
Durham, North Carolina

Lisa Liner, MD
Pediatric Resident
A.I. DuPont Hospital for Children
Wilmington, Delaware

Anagh Vora, MD
International Medical Graduate
Transitional Year Resident
St. Luke's Medical Center
Milwaukee, Wisconsin

Derek Wayman, MD
PGY-1, Family Practice Resident
University of North Dakota
Grand Forks, North Dakota

Marketa Wills, MD
Clinical Fellow, Psychiatry
Harvard Medical School
PGY-IV Chief Resident
Massachusetts General Hospital
Boston, Massachusetts

Preface

If you have reviewed the USMLE Step 3 Computer-Based Case Simulation (CCS) sample material and experimented with the computerized patients, you probably tried testing the limits of the software—perhaps you even tried giving a drug overdose or performing aggressive surgery. Whatever your method, the fact that you would take risks with a computerized patient that you would *never* take with a real one illustrates one of many differences between simulated and actual patient care. The CCS mimics real patient management; however, the pronounced differences between computerized and real patients may cause even an excellent physician and problem solver to struggle with this portion of the Step 3 exam.

Step 2 and Step 3 of the USMLE are both clinically based. Step 2 tests your ability to practice medicine while supervised, and Step 3 tests the knowledge needed for the unsupervised practice of medicine.[1] The multiple-choice questions are similar on both exams; after all, what you need to know to practice medicine doesn't change whether you are supervised or not. The most noticeable difference between Step 2 and Step 3 is the CCS—a complex, interactive test format designed to simulate real patient management. Most Step 3 review books concentrate on medical facts and provide no technical advice about the CCS, such as how to navigate the computer program. This CCS guide will supplement the review books you already have so you can be fully prepared for Step 3.

The CCS format is new and unfamiliar to Step 3 test-takers, and the guesswork involved with treating artificial patients can be frustrating. Fortunately, the uncertainty associated with the CCS can be overcome. In fact, this portion of the exam is easy if you familiarize yourself with the test format and learn how to apply your clinical knowledge effectively to the exam. This guide will:

- Clarify the exam format
- Offer general information about scheduling the exam
- Present a strategy for approaching your cases
- Discuss the CCS scoring process
- Teach you how to predict your specific case topics
- Provide several sample cases using the exam format

By the time you finish this book, you will know how to manage your computerized patients so you can focus on medicine, rather than on the intricacies of the testing software.

To get the most from this guide, practice with the CCS exam format before reading further. The concepts presented in the pages ahead will make more sense if you have experimented with the CCS before reading on. Practice cases are available on the USMLE website (http://www.usmle.org) and on an instructional CD that will be mailed to you by the examiners after you register for the test.

Good luck with your exam preparation!

1 Scheduling and Preparing for the Exam

In most cases, completing medical school adequately prepares you for Step 3. Nonetheless, many people have the false impression that an additional year of training will help them prepare for the exam. While the additional clinical training expands your specialty skills, your general medical knowledge and test-taking aptitude may actually deteriorate somewhat over the year, depending on your chosen specialty. In addition to being more focused on their training, interns tend to be much busier—and therefore have less time to study—than senior medical students. If possible, prepare for the exam as a medical student and arrange to take the exam as soon as you can.

■ PRE-EXAM REQUIREMENTS

Complete Medical School and Pass USMLE Steps 1 and 2

You must pass the USMLE Step 1, Step 2 CK and Step 2 CS, and obtain a medical school diploma in order to register for the USMLE Step 3.

Post Medical School Training

State laws determine when you are allowed to take Step 3. Some states allow you to take the exam immediately after finishing medical school, whereas others require completion of one year of residency training prior to taking the exam. For a current list of state requirements for taking Step 3, visit http://www.fsmb.org.

State Medical Board Selection

When registering for Step 3, you must choose a state medical board to approve your exam. Each state has its own exam requirements, including when you can take it, how many attempts you are allowed to pass, and how the exam is tied to licensure. *You may select any state as your approving body, and schedule the exam under that state's requirements.* Shop around for a state whose rules fit your needs, and be sure that you understand that state's requirements fully before registering. You do not need to live or practice in the state you select to approve your exam. If you wish to take the exam immediately after finishing medical school, be sure to select a state that does not require one year of residency prior to taking the exam. Be sure to check with the medical board of the state you plan to have approve your exam for their current requirements.

■ EXAM PREPARATION

You may be familiar with the "Rule of Twos" for USMLE test preparation: Study two months for Step 1, two weeks for Step 2, and two days for Step 3. By the time most people are preparing to take Step 3, they have already secured their residency position and they use and promote the "Rule of Twos." Others feel that their clinical experience negates the need for rigorous study. Unfortunately, clinical experience has its limitations (in that general knowledge and test-taking skills may fade) and it certainly won't help prepare you for the complex CCS exam format. Additionally, everyone has weak points in his or her knowledge of clinical medicine. Studying for the USMLE provides the perfect opportunity to review the skills needed for proper patient care in any field of medicine. A little focused preparation will enable you to obtain the best possible score and learn from the exam, which benefits you and, ultimately, your patients.

■ ADVICE FOR INTERNATIONAL MEDICAL GRADUATES

Exam preparation and the challenges of the CCS may be intensified for international medical graduates (IMGs) for a variety of reasons, such as the following:

- Compared to U.S. medical school graduates, IMGs often take the USMLE series at different intervals and at different points in their careers. Some take all the USMLE steps at once, years after their medical school training.

- To U.S. medical training program directors, IMGs may have a less certain training background, and are therefore more likely to be evaluated primarily by their USMLE scores.

- The standard of care for many illnesses varies throughout the world. The USMLE and CCS cases are scored according to the U.S. standards of medical practice. People who did not train in the United States must become familiar with U.S. standards, for both the exam and medical practice.

The obstacles for IMGs can be overcome. The best time to take the USMLE series is highly individual. Because the Step 2 and Step 3 multiple-choice questions are quite similar, reviewing once and taking both exams without delay may be the best strategy. It is important, however, to allow sufficient time between tests in order to become familiar with the CCS. This book will streamline your CCS preparation because it is specifically designed to familiarize the reader with the types of cases that will be tested and the depth of patient management required to perform adequately. A test-taker's clinical experience and training background may vary considerably depending on where he or she trained, and becoming familiar with the U.S. standards of medical practice is critical for scoring well on the USMLE and becoming a competent physician in the United States. Compared to medical practice abroad, U.S. medical practice may differ not only by test and treatment characteristics, but also by patients' attitudes and beliefs about what is appropriate in a given medical setting. The USMLE Steps 2 and 3 both contain numerous questions about what represents an appropriate verbal response to a patient in a given situation. The following suggestions will help prepare IMGs:

- Spend time in a U.S. hospital—this is probably the best way to become familiar with the U.S. practice of medicine in terms of medical facts and cultural differences in the patient population.

- Use a general USMLE review book well in advance of taking the exams to help you identify the parts of your medical background, if any, that differ from U.S. practice standards.

- Rotate through general medical fields like internal medicine or family practice for an overall exposure, and choose specific fields (like radiology or intensive care) if you find your background differs from the U.S. practice standards.

By following the above suggestions, you will learn medical facts according to U.S. standards and adjust to the way patients in the United States feel about their medical care.

2 Conquering the CCS

The CCS consists of a series of patients with differing medical problems that you must manage. Having a consistent strategy for each case will increase your effectiveness significantly. The strategy presented here allows you to formulate your treatment approach quickly, and helps prevent you from panicking if your computerized patient's health doesn't improve after your initial efforts.

Each case begins with an introductory statement about the patient followed by their vital signs and history. After reading the introduction, consider each case in two stages:

1. The *initial management stage* consists of the physical exam and numerous orders and actions that address the acute medical problem.
2. The *watching and waiting stage* consists of monitoring your patient while your initial actions take effect.

This two-stage approach can be applied to every case, although the order is somewhat interchangeable. For instance, in an emergency, you may provide some initial treatment before examining the patient or ordering tests. To implement the strategy, consider the steps outlined in Box 2.1 as you work through each case.

The following is a detailed breakdown of each step in the strategy:

■ 1. INITIAL MANAGEMENT STAGE

1a. Reading the Introductory Statement and Patient History

The opening lines of each case form your initial impression of the patient, and his or her history provides the basic information necessary to plan your treatment approach. Remember that this

BOX 2.1	10 STEP CCS STRATEGY

1. Initial Management

   1a. Read the introductory statement and patient history

   1b. Take notes about the case

   1c. Determine the treatment location

   1d. Perform the physical exam

   1e. Formulate a differential diagnosis

   1f. Order tests (to confirm your diagnosis)

   1g. Determine the treatment location (again!)

   1h. Provide treatment

2. Watching and Waiting

   2a. Address secondary problems (using the notes you took in step 1b)

   2b. Set follow-up appointments/Advance the clock

exam tests general medical knowledge and patient management skills; therefore, each patient's presenting complaint will probably be straightforward and highly suggestive of his or her diagnosis. In reality, you were likely taught to consider rare diseases and unusual patient presentations. However, applying this reasoning to the exam may actually lead you away from the common conditions being tested. Your first impression about your patient's diagnosis is probably correct.

1b. Taking Notes

You must step away from the patient's major medical problem for a moment and extract some information for later in the case. Almost every patient will have problems that aren't part of his or her major presenting complaint. For example, a patient complaining of chest pain may be overweight, unemployed, or homeless. These secondary problems, in addition to the primary medical problem, must be addressed to provide optimal care. Unfortunately, in the simulation many cases will abruptly end in the middle (case ending is addressed in Chapter 3, Managing Time), allowing you to only add or delete orders without reviewing the patient's record. Secondary problems are easily forgotten unless you make a note of them early in the case. You will be given a dry erase board and marker to use during your exam. Use these to take notes as you read a patient's history. Jot down a word or two about each potential secondary problem as you encounter it in the case presentation. A sample list may be: "obese, smokes, unemployed." For cases that continue after your initial treatment, you can review the patient's history for cues. For cases that end abruptly, you will be able to review the notes you made and provide treatment or advice for these secondary problems. You *must* address the patient's primary medical problem first; for now you are just taking notes. More information about addressing these secondary problems is provided in Section 2, Watching and Waiting.

1c. Determining the Treatment Location

After reading a patient's introductory statement and history, select the best initial treatment location for the patient. Your location choices include the patient's home, your office, the emergency room, the hospital ward, and the intensive care unit. The majority of your cases will originate in your office or the emergency room. In reality, you know where you are treating your patient and whether the location is appropriate, but on the exam, all simulated settings appear the same. *Because you cannot physically see your computerized patient or his or her surroundings, it is easy to begin treating a patient without concern for the setting.* You must specifically plan to address the patient's treatment location so that you don't begin a lengthy workup in the original location, which may be inappropriate. For example, you may realize well into the case that you have been treating a patient for a week in the emergency room. You must then decide whether to abruptly change the location or to continue treatment in the wrong setting. Although changing location in the middle of the case seems unrealistic and may make you feel like you are mismanaging the case, your orders will stand and the course of treatment will remain the same in the new location. Therefore, if you initially forget to address the location, it is better to change location late than to continue treatment in the wrong place. Plan to assess treatment location at the beginning of each case, and then again after the patient's condition evolves. The proper initial location depends on the information presented in the introductory statement and history.

1d. Performing the Physical Exam

The CCS physical exam is easy to perform and the results are very thorough. You have the option of performing a complete exam, or you can save time by selecting only the specific organ systems you wish to examine. If your patient is unstable for any reason you should perform a very focused physical exam and start treatment immediately. However, you must take the necessary time to accurately assess each patient. The balance between being complete and being fast can be delicate for unstable patients. Let your clinical experience be your guide.

Note that you must *always* perform a complete physical exam for each patient, even if you start with a focused physical exam. *The CCS tests your ability to provide proper general medical care*, which includes performing a thorough physical examination of each patient. If necessary, focus your exam initially, but always perform a full physical exam at some point in the case. Also, do not forget to examine your patient periodically throughout the case. You may conduct a physical exam once and become so involved in treatment that you forget to reexamine the patient. Obtain an interval history and physical exam either daily or every time a patient's condition changes. Your daily exams may be focused to save time, but you should continue them as part of your patient's care.

1e. Formulating a Differential Diagnosis

Once again, remember that this is a general medical exam and your patients will present with the typical features of common medical problems. Pursuing rare diseases or unusual presentations may lead you astray on this exam. Formulating a simple differential diagnosis will help you determine which tests to order and how you should interpret their results.

1f. Ordering Tests

The specifics of each case dictate which tests are appropriate. *As a rule, start conservatively.* Excessive lab tests and procedures waste time and will count against you (see Chapter 5, Scoring), but the proper diagnosis of each patient is imperative. If you begin with a solid differential diagnosis you will know what you are testing for and won't be confused by negative or unexpected test results. However, an unexpected result can be very informative and doesn't necessarily mean the test was ordered erroneously. If you do get an unexpected test result, first try to determine why by reassessing your differential diagnosis, and then move forward. It is better to order a few extra tests and promptly reach a diagnosis than to allow your concern for overordering delay prompt subsequent management.

Ordering tests is a crucial part of the exam and practicing your orders will benefit you greatly. When ordering tests, remember the following:

- After ordering a test, the results are stored in a file accessible at the top of the screen. You can review your entire interaction with a patient at any time during the case by clicking on the tabs located near the top of the screen. There are individual tabs labeled "Order Sheet," "Progress Notes," "Vital Signs," "Lab Reports," "Imaging," "Other Tests," and "Treatment Record" that organize the tests and treatments you have performed.

- On the CCS, tests are interpreted for you. If you order an x-ray or an ECG, *you do not have to read it.* A complete interpretation is provided.

- The normal range of lab values is reported with the results of any lab test you order. *You do not have to memorize normal lab values or search through a list of normal values.*

- Do not try to budget sleep hours for you or your patient on the exam. Order tests and begin treatment as soon as possible, even if the setting is late at night and you would wait until morning in reality.

1g. Determining the Treatment Location (Again!)

To avoid the frustration of realizing halfway through the case that your patient is in the wrong location, plan to reevaluate the patient's location again at a later point. Once you receive test results and have made a diagnosis, it may be necessary to relocate your patient. Reconsider the location any time a significant change occurs in your patient's care.

1h. Providing Treatment

After reviewing the test results and ensuring that your patient is in the proper location, you may begin providing treatment. You may have treated an emergent condition or symptom like pain initially, but now you must provide definitive medical intervention for your patient's ailment. When ordering treatments, consider the following:

- During treatment, the patient or a family member may spontaneously update you. For example, a message may suddenly appear on the screen saying that your patient's condition has improved (or deteriorated) after your initial effort. These messages do not necessarily mean that you should change the way you are managing the case. Your patient may complain of pain despite proper treatment, or the pain may diminish while the patient remains in critical condition. These remarks are not meant to provide hints or lead you astray; they are merely intended to simulate a real patient's remarks. *Although you may be tempted to compensate immediately if a patient complains, let your knowledge of how a real patient might respond guide your treatment strategy.*

- On the exam you play the role of a general practitioner. In some cases, you may need to consult a specialist for a complex problem or surgery. When requesting a consult, you must order the specific consultant (pulmonary consult, surgery consult, etc.) and provide justification. You will never be denied a consultation based on your justification. Also, unlike reality, a CCS consultant will never provide any meaningful advice. The exam is testing *you*, and the consultants won't provide advice as they do in reality. *Therefore, you should never consult a specialist because you don't know what to do with your patient.* You will be unable to justify your request adequately and your consultant will only tell you that you must continue to manage your patient as needed. Order consults only to document your request for the sake of scoring, not to obtain advice about your patient.

- You will encounter at least one patient who requires surgical intervention, and you must know how to order surgery. After determining that your patient requires surgery, request a surgical consult. Be specific with your request (general surgery, thoracic surgery, etc.). Remember, the surgical consultant will see your patient but will not provide advice. Perform the necessary preoperative measures (antibiotics, NPO, IV fluids, etc.), and directly order the *specific* surgical procedure (e.g., appendectomy or splenectomy, etc.) your patient requires. If you want the procedure done laparoscopically, you must specify that as well.

- Delivering a baby works the same way as ordering surgery. When it is necessary to deliver, request an obstetric consult first, then order the delivery directly.

- If you forget to request a consultation before you order surgery, a reminder will appear on your screen and you will be required to request consultation first.

- If you order fluids for a patient, you will be required to specify what kind. Order normal saline, lactated Ringer solution, or "keep vein open" if you want venous access and fluid loss or retention is not a consideration. If managing fluid overload or loss is part of the case, typing "fluids" in the order form will bring up a long list of different fluids for you to select from based on your patient's needs. You are not required to give a rate of fluid administration.

- Medication orders do not require doses, and you cannot change the amount given. You are, however, required to specify the route of administration for example, by vein (IV) or by mouth (PO), and so on . . . and whether the drug is to be administered once or continuously. Both generic and name brand medication orders are recognized.

As you work though the initial management, concentrate on progressing from one step to the next (steps 1a-1h). Because each case is timed, you may feel pressure to solve your patient's problems all at once. Your successes will come intermittently as you work through the diagnosis and treatment of each patient. Utilizing this eight-step approach for initial patient management will put you in control and increase your efficiency on the exam.

■ 2. WATCHING AND WAITING

2a. Addressing Secondary Problems

After you have performed the immediately necessary tests and treatments, some cases will end abruptly. You will know the case is ending when a box appears on screen telling you to finalize your care for the patient. There is no way to tell beforehand when a case will end or which cases will end before you are finished. Cases that end early are testing your initial approach to the patient. Cases that continue beyond your first effort are testing your initial approach and your ability to follow up on the care you provided. You must learn to take advantage of any extra time you are given with a patient.

Step 1b of the initial management stage reminded you to take notes about the patient's minor health or social problems as you encountered them in the history. After a patient's primary medical problem has been treated, it is time to address the patient's secondary problems. These problems are usually mentioned briefly in the patient history and are often completely unrelated to the patient's acute medical condition. Almost all of your patients will have at least one secondary condition that requires attention. To disregard these needs is to provide less than optimal patient care. If you treat the patient's primary concern and the case hasn't ended, start by returning to the initial information you received about your patient. The patient's history and physical exam findings often contain significant—but easily overlooked—secondary problems. If the computer program ends the case abruptly, allowing you to only type new orders and not review the patient's chart, you will have the notes you took at the beginning of the case to help you remember your patient's secondary problems. Most of these problems can be handled through counseling, patient education, or social work. Typing "counsel" or "educate" in the order form will bring up an extensive list of subjects. Each patient will undoubtedly need advice on one of the subjects listed. Ordering "counseling" or "education" on the subject of concern is all that is needed (for the purpose of scoring) to show that you considered your patient's needs beyond the acute medical problem.

During the watching and waiting phase, you should also consider your patients' health maintenance, including vaccines and screening tests, as secondary concerns. In reality, this important part of patient care is usually completed at preset time intervals. Considering health maintenance procedures for your computerized patients can be tricky because you often don't know when the patient's next procedure or test is due. In Chapter 5, Scoring, you will learn that some orders may count against you if they are timed inappropriately for a given patient. For example, a patient presenting with acute chest pain may also be due for a Pap smear. If you order a Pap smear, the computer may interpret your order as an inappropriate treatment for a heart attack rather than the health maintenance measure you intended. Additionally, ordering vaccines for a child based on age alone is irresponsible. *To avoid confusion, order health maintenance procedures only for those patients who definitely need them.* This includes patients who have a documented, outdated procedure (Pap smear, vaccine, etc.) listed in their history and those who do not receive frequent health care, such as the homeless. Only consider ordering a health maintenance test or procedure after the patient's acute medical condition has been appropriately addressed.

2b. Setting Follow-up Appointments/Advancing the Clock

You must schedule follow-up appointments and learn how to advance the clock as part of the Watching and Waiting stage. The appropriate follow-up for each patient will vary depending on the circumstances. To learn more about scheduling follow-up and advancing the clock, please see Chapter 3, Managing Time.

3 Managing Time

Having to advance the clock is probably the computer simulation's greatest deviation from reality. Learning to manage the clock can be difficult, and mastering it before taking the exam is essential. In each case there are two times to be aware of:

1. *Real time*—the time that is passing while you take the exam.
2. *Simulated time*—the time that passes for your patient, his or her disease, and your treatment.

During your initial management of each case, the real and simulated times are roughly equal. As you begin waiting for results or scheduling follow-up appointments, the simulated time can stretch into days and weeks. The amount of simulated time needed for follow-up and treatment will differ in each case.

During the test there are two digital clocks at the bottom of your computer screen. One clock shows the elapsed real time and the other shows the elapsed simulated time. Additionally, there is a clock face on the top of the screen with an hour and minute hand that rotate as the simulated time passes. The computer also tells you how much simulated time each procedure or order will take after you have requested it. It is not necessary to be as aware of simulated time as these features imply you should be. If you are watching that clock and trying to account for each passing hour, you are becoming too concerned about the simulated time. *In fact, simulated time doesn't really matter except in emergent cases when death is imminent.* If you are managing your patient correctly, the simulated time will pass appropriately without your concern. There is a lot to concentrate on in each case and you can safely ignore the simulated time except in the direst emergencies.

■ ADVANCING THE CLOCK

There are several ways to minimize the confusion associated with simulated time and having to advance the clock. When you choose to advance the clock you must click on the clock face on the top of the computer screen labeled "Obtain Results or See Patient Later." A window will appear with a calendar and a choice to reevaluate the patient in one of four ways:

- on (a specified time)
- in (a specified amount of time)
- with next available result
- call/see me as needed

When waiting for results in the initial management phase, use the "with next available result" option only. This option is difficult to adjust to because the real-life equivalent is absurd: waiting in the lab for your patient's test results. On the exam, however, you treat one patient at a time, and he or she is your only concern. The "with next available result" option is best because it is easy to use and you are automatically made aware of your patient's results as soon as they become available. The alternative, scheduling your next call using the "on" or "in" option, requires you to select a time and date from the calendar. You must then note the amount of time the test will take and arrange to be called sometime after that. It is not wrong to use these options, but they require much more planning on your part. Using the "next available result" option during the initial management gets you timely results and keeps you from being distracted with scheduling your next call.

As a case progresses to the watching and waiting stage, you may need to schedule an appointment or daily visits. You should then use the "on" or "in" option with the calendar to do so. When scheduling follow-up, you can afford to be a lot less punctual than you must be when awaiting a critical lab result. Using the "on" or "in" option before it is necessary creates extra work for you and should be avoided until the circumstances require you to schedule your visits with your patient.

Using the "call/see me as needed option" implies that you are done with the patient and the case. Often your patient will give you an update about his or her condition after you select this option. Based on the update, you can reconsider and see your patient, or you can continue advancing the clock using the "call/see me as needed" option until the case ends. The patient's condition and your experience will tell you whether it is necessary to reevaluate the patient.

■ COMPLETING A CASE

The way in which the cases end is a source of confusion for many test-takers. As mentioned previously, you are often cut off from a case in the middle, with test results pending and treatment in progress. When a case is over, a box appears on screen instructing you to delete or add orders that are relevant to your patient's care. *You cannot go back to your patient at this point.* How are you supposed to know what a patient will need under these circumstances? What treatments can be stopped? Does the case ending imply that your patient has died or has been sent home? Imagine the case cut off as a moment in time during your patient's care. Your patient and his or her disease are frozen where they are when the case ends. You should not assume that your patient and his or her illness continue to evolve in any way. If you were about to order or cancel something, you should still do so, but you should not stop an ongoing treatment or schedule a follow-up appointment because you are in the middle of providing care for your patient. You should also not schedule a future test or treatment unless you know it is necessary. A test or order that may be appropriate later in the case is not necessarily appropriate when you are cut off, and shouldn't be ordered. *Don't order everything you think the patient may eventually need.* Using this logic, you might then have to cancel those orders because your patient will eventually get better and not require them. You'd be in a useless cycle predicting how the patient's health will evolve and making and canceling orders. When a case ends you have either already demonstrated or not demonstrated your ability for the purpose of scoring that case. For example, a case may be testing your initial management of chest pain. Very soon after the case starts, your initial management becomes obvious and the case will end. Your first responses were either right or wrong, and you will be scored accordingly. How you would have followed up with the patient was not a testing point of that case, so the fact that the case ended early doesn't matter. When a case stops abruptly, simply make your very next move and confidently let the case end wherever you are in the course of your management.

CCS versus Reality

The strategy outlined in Chapter 2, Conquering the CCS, provides a focused approach to the medical management component of each case. For the most part, providing actual medical care such as ordering tests and treatments and getting results in the computer simulation is a good approximation of reality. Unfortunately, there are aspects of the exam that are confusing and do not directly relate to medical management or accurately reflect real patient care. For example, having to choose the best location for treatment without being able to see the patient is not very realistic. The exam instructions direct you to behave on the exam exactly as you would in reality, but also present several realistic orders and actions that cannot be carried out in the simulation. Test-takers are often left wondering how close their simulated actions should represent real patient care.

■ HOW REALISTIC IS THE CCS?

You can perform the significant components of medical management (e.g., physical exams, treatments, medications, etc.) just as you would for an actual patient. However, there are many important orders that apply to real patients that may not be practical in the computer simulation. For example, when presented with your virtual patient, you can make an order requesting his or her past medical record. While this constitutes routine patient care in reality, is it necessary or useful on the exam? Unless the history specifically states the patient is making a return visit, you never actually receive a prior medical record on the exam. However, the order is among those the computer recognizes and reflects a level of completeness in patient management.

The computer also recognizes the order "Reassure patient." In reality, you probably reassure your patients at every visit. On the exam, you have limited time to complete each case. You don't want to continuously order reassurance for your patient in lieu of providing medical intervention. The computer's recognition of certain detailed orders and its failure to recognize others creates a problem for those striving for an outstanding score and thorough patient management. *The exam is not a perfect simulation, and you must deviate from reality.* Because this is true, the question is, by how much? To what level of reality are you held responsible? The exam instructions do not address these questions specifically, and only offer the suggestion that some detailed orders, such as diet and ambulation, receive little weight unless they are somehow essential to the patient's care. However, ordering appropriate screening tests that are not essential to the patient's acute medical care are accounted for in your overall exam performance. You don't want to be left guessing which orders are important and which are not. You want to manage each patient impeccably, and let those scoring the exam determine what is important.

You can learn to approximate reality best on the exam by becoming familiar with the types of commands the test software will recognize. By learning which orders the computer will accept, you will develop a feel for how closely your management must approximate reality. When a specific situation arises, you can then decide whether to pursue the details, or stick to the main points and move on. The list of orders in Box 4.1 represents a small sample of commands the computer recognizes. Some of these orders were selected because they are easily forgotten. Others are things you may informally mention to a patient in reality, but not actually order in the patient's medical record as you must on the exam. Using these orders when appropriate may add a level of completeness to your patient management.

These examples are provided so you do not overlook certain details when managing your computerized patients. Some are also easy to forget while focusing on more critical tests and treatments during this timed exam. Use the sample CCS cases on the practice CD or USMLE website to experiment with these and similar orders until you get a sense of the things the computer will recognize. For instance, try ordering a pizza just to see how the computer responds.

BOX 4.1	UNUSUAL AND EASILY OVERLOOKED ORDERS RECOGNIZED BY THE CCS

Medical record request	Bathe patient
Isolation	Comfort patient
Social work consult	Reassure patient
Restrain patient	Limit caffeine/alcohol
Wound dressing	Sun screen
Bandage wound	Medication compliance
Bathroom privileges	Council (brings up a large list of options)
Child protective services consult	
NPO	Educate (brings up a large list of options)
Absence note from school or work	
Treat sex partner	Precautions (brings up a large list of options)
Home glucose monitoring	
Caution (brings up a large list of options)	Cane
	Walker
Pulse oximetry	Call physician if suicidal
Advance directive	Vitamins
Living will	Consent for procedure
Transfuse blood	Transcendental meditation

■ GENERAL TIPS ON ORDERING

Orders are made by clicking the "Order Sheet" tab on the top of the computer screen. This brings up a list of the orders you have made, if any, and allows you to make new orders by selecting the "Order" box at the bottom of the screen. If you select "Order," a blank order form will appear that allows you to type in your order. After typing, you must click on the "Confirm Order" tab. You can write several orders at once by pressing the enter key after each order. You can then click "Confirm Order" only once instead of after each order. *Doing this will save you the extra time required to reselect the "Order Sheet" tab and wait for the computer to process each order individually.* As you become familiar with making orders, you may discover that many orders can be abbreviated. If you type the first three letters of an order, the computer will either recognize it or give you the option to choose among similarly worded commands. Using the order form this way allows you to broaden your options. By making a general or abbreviated order, you force the computer to generate a list of orders from which you can choose. You may find an order that is better for your patient than the one you originally intended to use. For example, if you believe your patient needs alcohol counseling, you will get many more related treatment options by typing just "alcohol" or "counseling" than you would by typing the entire command.

Making the computer generate lists produces a frightening number of different orders, some you may not even recognize. Don't worry; this does not imply that patient management will be overly demanding or complex. USMLE test-takers are diverse in their abilities, training, and backgrounds. To accurately assess each test-taker's skill, the exam must be able to accommodate all levels of expertise. Remember, almost all of the cases consist of basic medical problems that can be managed using the routine tests and treatments you are already familiar with.

Scoring

In spite of the importance of passing the USMLE, little information about the scoring process is readily available. Obviously, the more multiple-choice questions you answer correctly, the better your score. Beyond that, the scaled scoring system used for the USMLE steps is elusive. The scoring of the CCS component of Step 3 is even less intuitive given the number of different ways each patient can be managed. Unfortunately, the exam's purpose and value as a measuring tool depends entirely on the final score. After hours of anguish and intense preparation, test-takers receive only a brief report and an ambiguous three-digit score. How are scoring errors detected? How is the test-taker supposed to learn from the exam? A great deal of information about the scoring process can be obtained beyond that provided in your score report.

Not all test-takers get the same multiple-choice questions or CCS topics, and some exams are probably somewhat more difficult than others. The raw score is the number of questions an examinee actually answered correctly. USMLE scores are reported as a scaled score. The scaled score is a manipulation of the raw score that accounts for varying question difficulty and allows a direct comparison among all exams. For example, someone who did well on an easy question block would get the same scaled score as someone answering fewer questions correctly on a more difficult block. The scaled score for Step 3 combines the multiple-choice and CCS scores. Scoring for each portion of the exam differs and will be discussed separately.

■ MULTIPLE-CHOICE SCORING

In the multiple-choice portion of the exam, each question is of equal value in determining the score. The total score is based on the number of questions answered correctly. There is no penalty

■ **TABLE 5.1**	
Sample Exam Scoring	
Question Number	**Chance of Correct Answer**
1	.65
2	.70
3	.50
4	.65
5	.50
Total	3.0

for guessing. Approximately 10 percent of questions on USMLE exams are trial questions. These questions are being pilot-tested for future use and are not used in tabulating the final scaled score.[2]

The minimum passing score is established using the modified Angoff standard setting procedure.[1] This process involves a group of experts (in this case, medical educators) who independently estimate the likelihood that a marginal student would answer each exam question correctly. These estimates are summed and the average number across the group of experts becomes the lowest passing score. In the example above, an expert determines (by guessing) that there is a 65 percent chance that a marginal student would answer question 1 correctly. The chance of a correct answer for each question, as determined by one expert, is shown in Table 5.1.

In the above five-question example, this scoring expert would recommend a passing score of 3 based on his or her perceived difficulty level of each question. Passing scores are determined by several experts in the same way and are then averaged to eliminate individual bias. This average becomes the passing raw score. This method, along with the use of trial questions as mentioned above, is presumably how questions and question blocks are assigned difficulty levels.

■ CCS SCORING

The CCS tests the timing and appropriateness of medical decision making in the absence of the artificial prompts inherent in multiple-choice questions. Scoring for the CCS portion of the exam is more complex because of its freeform nature. This unique testing format requires a specialized scoring system derived from a computer program called CBX (Computer-Based Examination).

In managing each case, the examinee generates a list of interactions, tests, and treatments for the patient. A record of these encounters is kept as a "transaction list" that shows what was ordered, when it was ordered, and when the test-taker received the results. The decision process used by the examinee in each case is elicited by the initial orders and the successive actions made after the result of each test or treatment becomes known. The CBX program converts the transaction list into a numerical score record.[3] A score for each case is generated by comparing the examinee's score record to a score key derived from experts in the following way.[4]

Experts are enlisted to produce a scoring key for each case by managing the case individually. Numerous experts compare their responses, agree on which orders or actions represent ideal management for that case, and classify them as either "good," "irrelevant," "bad," or "failure." Box 5.1 describes the four possible classifications for each action/order.

Points are then assigned to each category: beneficial orders/actions count as positive points (the more appropriate the order, the more points awarded), irrelevant orders have no value, and

---

BOX 5.1	CCS ORDER SCORING KEY

GOOD: Essential for proper patient care

IRRELEVANT: Unnecessary, but not harmful to the patient

BAD: Potentially risky to patient

FAILURE: Excessively risky to the patient or demonstrates total misunderstanding of the case objective

bad orders/actions subtract from the score. The value of each beneficial order is then weighted based on timeliness, importance to patient care, and difficulty (how likely a test-taker is to remember to perform that order). Irrelevant orders delay beneficial orders and probably indirectly count against you. The CBX program compares an examinee's score record to the ideal and minimal passing score set by the cumulative opinion of the experts. This process effectively simulates the scoring as it would be if a group of experts interpreted and scored each test-taker's responses individually.[5]

The final USMLE test score is derived from an examinee's combined performance on the CCS and multiple-choice question portions of the exam. Determining the extent to which each component contributes to the final score is complex. The CCS and multiple-choice questions measure a physician's ability somewhat differently, and the proportion of each component on the test and the test length determine the effectiveness of the exam.[5] Numerous weighting methods have been described, and exams with more than one format are frequently weighted by the time allotted for each.[6] As such, the CCS component comprises 25 percent of the exam time and probably accounts for close to 25 percent of the final score.

Sample Cases

Although the list of potential case topics is seemingly limitless, you can anticipate the subject of your cases better than you may think. Even though there are multiple versions of the USMLE exams, the following can be said about your exam with near certainty:

- You will have a patient requiring surgical intervention
- You will have a patient with chest pain
- You will have a patient with an infectious disease
- You will have more than one patient with common, acute, or chronic medical problems
- You will **not** have a patient requiring an extensive cancer workup
- You will **not** have a patient with a psychiatric illness
- You will **not** have a patient requiring a controversial or very new treatment or procedure
- You will **not** have a patient in need of a general checkup who has no specific complaints

■ PREDICTING YOUR CASE TOPICS

Once again remember that this exam is meant to test general medical concepts. This fact is evident in the practice CCS cases provided by the examiners. The specific diseases represented in the practice cases may not appear on your exam, but the general skills needed to manage them will be the same. Using the concepts inherent in the practice cases, you can predict specific illnesses that are likely to appear on your exam. *A medical problem that requires some basic clinical knowledge, a few commonly used diagnostic skills, and a treatment that isn't controversial is the perfect exam case*. Managing a myocardial infarct, for instance, requires a good differential diagnosis, several diagnostic tests, and a widely accepted treatment. It is a great subject for the exam. Cancer, by contrast, requires treatment that is highly patient-specific and a significant workup involving many medical specialties. It is not a realistic exam topic. Psychiatric illness is difficult to convey in a computer simulation and also requires highly individualized care; it is therefore also probably not a good exam topic. As you go through your review books, certain diseases will seem fitting as potential case subjects because they have the above-mentioned characteristics. Write them down and review them again on the evening before the exam. Following these guidelines will provide structure to your CCS review, and allow you to predict the subject of many of your cases before the exam.

■ SAMPLE CASES

The following fifteen cases are common medical conditions and have patient presentation, diagnostic, and treatment characteristics that make them good exam topics. They are presented in the format that is outlined in this guide and used on the exam. Each case is designed to approximate the CCS in subject matter and difficulty as closely as possible, but there are some differences between the following cases and what you may encounter on the exam. First, each case is presented in the order of the strategy outlined in Chapter 2 (i.e., physical exam first, then ordering tests, then providing treatment). Many of your cases on the exam will follow this order, but some may not. For example, in an emergency it may be better to provide treatment before waiting for all the test results or completing the physical exam. Second, to keep the following cases simple, normal test results or physical exam findings are either not reported or reported as "normal." On the exam, when a test result or physical exam finding is normal you will get a description of what is normal, and must then interpret it as such. The exam may also have more lengthy patient histories than what is presented here. Finally, each case has a potential cut-off point designed to mimic the abrupt way your cases will end on the exam. In the following cases, the cut-off point always occurs after treatment has been rendered. On the exam, the cases can end at any time. While these cases represent typical case topics and the depth of knowledge required for the exam, do not be surprised if the computer-based simulation cases on the exam are a bit more dynamic than what is allowed by the rigid format necessary to portray them on paper. In order to get the most out of the sample cases you should:

- Cover the page as you read and introduce yourself to the cases line by line
- Test yourself by deciding what you would do at each step before looking ahead
- Remember that there are a number of appropriate ways to handle most medical problems.

What follows is by no means inclusive of the diseases you may see on your test. These topics are meant to provide a start to your review and demonstrate the level of knowledge you need to effectively manage each case.

CASE 1

Initial Presentation and Contributing History: A 64-year-old male comes to your office complaining of a gradual onset of fever, chills, and a productive cough.

Vital Signs:

Temp: 39°C (102.2°F)	BP systolic: 135 mmHg
Pulse: 84 beats/min; regular rhythm	BP diastolic: 86 mmHg
Respiratory rate: 22/min	Height: 183 cm (72 in)
	Weight: 110 kg (242 lbs)

The symptoms began two days ago. He has a cough producing thick, yellow sputum that is occasionally blood-tinged. He reports mild pain over his left posterior chest with deep inspiration. The patient smokes and has a history of chronic obstructive pulmonary disease. He was in a car accident 20 years ago that required a splenectomy. The rest of the history is noncontributory. *(Reminder: make your list now.)*

Patient Location: The best initial location depends on the severity of the symptoms. If the patient is comfortably breathing at rest, the office is probably okay for now. If the patient is very short of breath, the emergency room would be a more appropriate initial setting, and you should transfer the patient immediately.

Physical Exam: The patient is stable, so do a complete physical exam. On exam he is coughing and appears ill. He has late inspiratory wheezes diffusely and dullness to percussion and decreased breath sounds over the left lung base. The rest of the exam is normal.

CASE 1 (continued)·

Differential Diagnosis: Pneumonia, upper respiratory infection, tuberculosis, congestive heart failure, pulmonary embolus, asthma

Order Tests:

> Complete blood count (CBC) (order as routine)
>
> Chest x-ray (CXR) (order as routine)
>
> Sputum Gram stain (order as routine)
>
> Sputum culture (order as routine)

Use the "call with next available result" option after you've ordered the tests, and begin treatment as soon as you have enough information to do so.

Test Results:

> CBC: White cell count 17000/mm^3 (nl = 3500–10500)
>
> CXR: Normal mediastinum, left lower lobe infiltrate, no masses present
>
> Impression: Left lower lobe pneumonia
>
> Sputum Gram stain: Gram-positive diplococci
>
> Sputum culture results: Pending

DIAGNOSIS: COMMUNITY-ACQUIRED PNEUMONIA

Review Patient Location: The severity of the chest x-ray, symptoms, and co-morbid conditions determine whether hospitalization or home treatment is appropriate. Severe symptoms, advanced age, and multiple co-morbid conditions favor hospitalization. This patient could be sent home with treatment.

CASE 1 (continued)

Order Treatments:

> Cefuroxime (oral and continuous)

The case may cut off here or sooner. If it doesn't, continue with the following.

Secondary Orders: Use your list to recall that the patient is overweight, smokes, and has had a splenectomy. Educate the patient on smoking, obesity, and diet. For health maintenance, order a pneumococcal vaccine (given his history of having a splenectomy).

Advance Clock/Follow-up Appointment: Schedule the patient to return in 10 days. After that, you can use the "call/see me as needed" option for advancing the clock until the case ends.

CASE 2

Initial Presentation and Contributing History: A 25-year-old female presents to the emergency department with sharp right-sided pelvic pain and vaginal bleeding.

Vital Signs:

Temp: 37°C (98.6°F)	BP systolic: 104 mmHg
Pulse: 88 beats/min; regular rhythm	BP diastolic: 64 mmHg
Respiratory rate: 24/min	Height: 168 cm (66 in)
	Weight: 64 kg (141 lbs)

The pain began one day ago and has gradually gotten worse. Her last menstrual period eight weeks ago was normal. Her vaginal bleeding has been intermittent for the past week and has now become acutely worse. She also reports intermittent back pain over the past few days. She is sexually active and reports having numerous sexual partners in the recent past. She has a history of pelvic inflammatory disease. She denies being pregnant, but uses no specific birth control. The rest of the history is noncontributory. *(Reminder: make your list now.)*

Patient Location: The patient's problem is not yet well defined. The emergency department is the best location until her condition is better characterized.

Physical Exam: The patient's bleeding may be severe, so do a focused physical exam including general appearance, chest/lungs, heart/cardiovascular, abdomen, and genitalia. Complete the exam later. On exam she is pale and diaphoretic. She is tachycardic. She has mild abdominal distension and a palpable, soft, tender, right-sided adnexal mass. She has bright red blood and dark blood clots in her vagina. The rest of the exam is normal.

CASE 2 (continued)

Differential Diagnosis: Ectopic pregnancy, ruptured ovarian cyst, spontaneous abortion, acute appendicitis, acute pelvic inflammatory disease

Order Tests:

Orthostatic vitals (order as stat)

Complete blood count (CBC) (order as stat)

Type and crossmatch blood (order as stat)

Human chorionic gonadotropin (HCG) quantitative, serum (order as stat)

Ultrasound, transvaginal (order as stat)

Use the "call with next available result" option after you've ordered the tests, and begin treatment as soon as you know the diagnosis.

Test Results:

Orthostatic vitals: Supine pulse 87 and BP 110/66; upright pulse 110 and BP 94/62

CBC: Hemoglobin 7 g/dL (nl = 12–16); hematocrit 22% (nl = 36–46)

Blood type: A−

HCG: 2050 mIU/ml (nl = zero with no intrauterine pregnancy)

Transvaginal ultrasound: No intrauterine gestational sac, right adnexal mass, pelvic fluid

Impression: Probable ectopic pregnancy

DIAGNOSIS: RUPTURED ECTOPIC PREGNANCY

Review Patient Location: Patient stability determines the best location. This patient is unstable, and requires emergent intervention. Emergent surgery from the emergency department should be performed prior to admission to the hospital ward.

CASE 2 (continued)

Order Treatments:

> IV fluid (normal saline)
>
> NPO
>
> Cefazolin (IV and continuous)
>
> Transfuse packed red blood cells
>
> Consent for procedure
>
> Gynecologic consult
>
> Salpingectomy by laparotomy
>
> Rhogam (intramuscular and once)
>
> Morphine (IV and continuous)
>
> Iron therapy (oral and continuous)

The case may cut off here or sooner. If it doesn't, continue with the following.

Secondary Orders: Use your list to recall that the patient has multiple sex partners and prior pelvic inflammatory disease. Counsel the patient about safe-sex practices and future pregnancy risk.

Advance Clock/Follow-up Appointment: Keep the patient in the hospital until she has recovered from surgery. Schedule the patient to return in one week. A follow-up hemoglobin and HCG level would be appropriate. After that, you can use the "call/see me as needed" option for advancing the clock until the case ends.

CASE 3

Initial Presentation and Contributing History: An 18-year-old female is brought to the emergency department by her brother and sister for lethargy and confusion.

Vital Signs:

Temp: 38°C (100.4°F)	BP systolic: 102 mmHg
Pulse: 86 beats/min; regular rhythm	BP diastolic: 60 mmHg
Respiratory rate: 29/min	Height: 157 cm (62 in)
	Weight: 67 kg (148 lbs)

The patient's symptoms began two days ago. She is tired, easily confused, and "hasn't been herself lately." She has Down syndrome and type 1 diabetes mellitus and requires daily help from her siblings. She carried out her daily activities as usual until two days ago when she became incontinent to urine and increasingly confused. Her primary doctor changed her insulin regimen last week. She takes no alcohol or medications except insulin. The rest of the history is noncontributory. *(Reminder: make your list now.)*

Patient Location: Mental status changes could have life-threatening causes. She should remain in the emergency department until her condition is better characterized.

Physical Exam: The patient is stable, so do a complete physical exam. The patient is somnolent and confused. She is tachycardic and breathing rapidly and deeply. She appears dehydrated and has diffuse abdominal tenderness. She looks dirty and smells of urine. The rest of the exam is normal.

Differential Diagnosis: Diabetic ketoacidosis, infection, toxic ingestion, delirium

CASE 3 (continued)

Order Tests:

> Basic metabolic profile (Chem 7) (order as stat)
>
> Complete blood count (CBC) (order as stat)
>
> Urinalysis (UA) (order as stat)
>
> Arterial blood gasses (ABG) (order as stat)
>
> Glycated hemoglobin (HbA1c) (order as routine)
>
> Electrocardiogram (ECG) (order as stat)
>
> Ketones, serum (order as stat)

Use the "call with next available result" option after you've ordered the tests, and begin treatment as soon as you know the diagnosis.

Test Results:

> Chem 7: Glucose 312 mg/dL (nl = 70–110), sodium 132 mEq/L (nl = 136–145), potassium 3.9 mEq/L (nl = 3.5–5.0)
>
> CBC: White count 13000/mm^3 (nl = 3500–10500)
>
> UA: Positive urine glucose and ketones
>
> ABG: pH 7.13 (nl = 7.35–7.45), HCO_3 14 mEq/L (nl = 22–28), $PaCO_2$ 36 mmHg (nl = 35–45)
>
> HbA1c 8.8% (nl<6.5)
>
> ECG: Regular rhythm, normal QRS complexes, normal ST waves
>
> Interpretation: Normal ECG
>
> Ketones, serum: Positive

DIAGNOSIS: DIABETIC KETOACIDOSIS

Review Patient Location: The patient's condition is life threatening and requires frequent monitoring. She should be treated in the intensive care unit.

CASE 3 (continued)

Order Treatments:

> Regular insulin (IV and continuous)
>
> IV fluids (normal saline)
>
> Potassium chloride (IV and continuous)
>
> Dextrose (IV and continuous when glucose gets below 250 mg/dl)
>
> Basic metabolic profile (Chem 7) (hourly)
>
> See patient every hour for interval/follow-up history

The case may cut off here or sooner. If it doesn't, continue with the following.

Secondary Orders: The patient and her family need to understand her disease and medication. Order a diabetic consult, diabetic diet, and diabetic teaching. Recall from your list that the patient's family was experiencing difficulties in managing her insulin and personal needs. Obtain a social work consult to evaluate her living arrangement and caretakers.

Advance Clock/Follow-up Appointment: When the patient's electrolytes are balanced and her symptoms are gone she can be discharged. Schedule the patient to see you in one week. After that, you can use the "call/see me as needed" option for advancing the clock until the case ends.

CASE 4

Initial Presentation and Contributing History: A 20-year-old male presents to the emergency room after falling while rock climbing four hours ago.

Vital Signs:

Temp: 37°C (98.6°F)	BP systolic: 98 mmHg
Pulse: 94 beats/min; regular rhythm	BP diastolic: 68 mmHg
Respiratory rate: 24/min	Height: 183 cm (72 in)
	Weight: 85 kg (187 lbs)

The otherwise healthy patient was rock climbing when he fell about 10 feet and landed on his left side. He had some abdominal pain initially. Since then, the pain has worsened and he now feels weak and tired. He reports no other injuries. The rest of the history is noncontributory. *(Reminder: make your list now.)*

Patient Location: The emergency department is the best place until the patient's injuries have been evaluated.

Physical Exam: The patient's condition appears to be worsening, so perform a focused physical exam including general appearance, chest/lungs, heart/cardiovascular, abdomen, extremities/spine, and neuro/psych. Complete the exam later. On exam, he is pale, alert, and oriented with no signs of head trauma. He has left upper quadrant abdominal pain and point tenderness over the left ninth and tenth ribs. An abrasion and faint ecchymosis are present over the left flank. The rest of the exam is normal.

Differential Diagnosis: Fractured ribs with splenic rupture

CASE 4 (continued)

Order Tests:

Orthostatic vitals (order as stat)

Complete blood count (CBC) (order as stat)

Computed tomography, abdomen (CT scan) (order as stat)

Type and crossmatch blood (order as stat)

Use the "call with next available result" option after you've ordered the tests, and begin treatment as soon as you know the diagnosis.

Test Results:

Orthostatic vitals: Supine pulse 85 and BP 112/68; upright pulse 105 and BP 96/62

CBC: Hemoglobin 7 g/dL (nl = 13–17); hematocrit 26% (nl = 40–52)

Abdominal CT scan: Splenic laceration, large perisplenic fluid collection, fractured ninth and tenth left ribs

Impression: Splenic rupture

Blood type: O–

DIAGNOSIS: SPLENIC RUPTURE

Review Patient Location: The patient requires immediate management of his ruptured spleen. Emergent surgery from the emergency department should be performed prior to admission to the hospital ward.

Order Treatments:

IV fluids (normal saline)

NPO

Cefazolin (IV and continuous)

Transfuse packed red blood cells

CASE 4 (continued)

Consent for procedure

General surgery consult

Splenectomy by laparotomy

Morphine (IV and continuous)

Bandage wound

The case may cut off here or sooner. If it doesn't, continue with the following.

Secondary Orders: Use your list to recall that the patient fell while rock climbing. Counsel the patient about safety. Order a pneumococcal vaccine for asplenic patients.

Advance Clock/Follow-up Appointment: Keep the patient in the hospital until he has recovered from surgery. Schedule a follow-up appointment one week after discharge. After that, you can use the "call/see me as needed" option for advancing the clock until the case ends.

CASE 5

Initial Presentation and Contributing History: A 6-year-old female is brought to your office by her mother for a cough, chest tightness, dyspnea, and wheezing.

Vital Signs:

Temp: 37°C (98.6°F)	BP systolic: 105 mmHg
Pulse: 102 beats/min; regular rhythm	BP diastolic: 76 mmHg
Respiratory rate: 28/min	Height: 115 cm (45 in)
	Weight: 20 kg (44 lbs)

The patient's symptoms began three hours ago. Similar, but less severe symptoms occur about four times a week. Her breathing is normal and she is active between episodes. Her symptoms worsen in the spring and fall and when she visits her father who is a smoker. She has a history of asthma requiring her to take albuterol twice daily. Her albuterol has run out and the girl's father has been giving her pills from an unlabeled bottle that haven't helped. The rest of the history is noncontributory. *(Reminder: make your list now.)*

Patient Location: Proper location depends on the severity of symptoms. Signs of impending respiratory arrest would require immediate transfer to the emergency department. Pulse oximetry or arterial blood gasses may help with the decision. Your office is a good location until you have examined this patient.

Physical Exam: The patient may need immediate treatment for respiratory failure, so perform a focused physical exam including general appearance, chest/lungs, and heart/cardiovascular. Complete the exam later. On exam the patient appears anxious. She is having difficulty breathing and speaking. She has supraclavicular retractions with inspiration and diffusely decreased breath sounds with inspiratory and expiratory wheezes. The rest of the exam is normal.

CASE 5 (continued)

Differential Diagnosis: Asthma, bronchiolitis, foreign body aspiration

Order Tests:

> Chest x-ray (CXR) (order as stat)
>
> Pulse oximetry (order as stat every hour)
>
> Peak expiratory flow (order as stat)
>
> Arterial blood gasses (ABG) (order as stat)

Use the "call with next available result" option after you've ordered the tests, and begin treatment as soon as you know the diagnosis.

Test Results:

> CXR: Hyperinflation and atelectasis, bones and heart normal, no foreign body
>
> Impression: Consistent with asthma
>
> Pulse oximetry: 91% (nl = 94–100)
>
> Peak expiratory flow: 100 L/min (nl = 215 L/min)
>
> ABG: pH 7.48 (nl = 7.35–7.45), $PaCO_2$ 26 mmHg (nl = 34–40), pO_2 67 mmHg (80–100), HCO_3: 21 mEq/L (nl = 22–28)

DIAGNOSIS: ASTHMA

Review Patient Location: The severity of this asthma attack (by peak expiratory flow and symptoms) warrants admission to the hospital ward.

Order Treatments:

> Oxygen (inhalation and continuous)
>
> Nebulized albuterol (inhalation and continuous)
>
> Methylprednisolone (IV and continuous)

CASE 5 (continued)

See the patient every hour until her symptoms improve. Send the patient home with a low-dose inhaled corticosteroid (beclomethasone) or a leukotriene antagonist (montelukast) for daily control of symptoms. Continue albuterol as needed.

The case may cut off here or sooner. If it doesn't, continue with the following.

Secondary Orders: Use your list to recall that the patient's father smokes and was giving her unlabeled pills. Educate the family about medication compliance and smoking.

Advance Clock/Follow-up Appointment: Schedule the patient to return in one week. After that, you can use the "call/see me as needed" option for advancing the clock until the case ends.

CASE 6

Initial Presentation and Contributing History: A 59-year-old male comes to your office complaining of pain in his fingers, knees, and hips.

Vital Signs:

Temp: 37°C (98.6°F)	BP systolic: 130 mmHg
Pulse: 70 beats/min; regular rhythm	BP diastolic: 76 mmHg
Respiratory rate: 22/min	Height: 183 cm (72 in)
	Weight: 93 kg (205 lbs)

The patient is a retired carpenter and has had progressively worsening pain at the base of his fingers on his right hand. Also, both knees and hips hurt when the patient stands for long periods of time. The symptoms have been present for about one year. He has no history of trauma to the joints. The pain keeps him sedentary, but he is generally healthy otherwise. The rest of the history is noncontributory. *(Reminder: make your list now.)*

Patient Location: There is no emergency, so the office is the best place.

Physical Exam: The patient is stable, so perform a complete physical exam. The patient is mildly overweight. He has slight quadriceps muscle atrophy bilaterally with crepitus and pain with motion of the knee and hip joints on both sides. There is no joint instability. There is mild tenderness of the metacarpophalangeal joints of his right hand. There are no Heberden or Bouchard nodes. The rest of the exam is normal.

Differential Diagnosis: Osteoarthritis, rheumatoid arthritis

CASE 6 (continued)

Order Tests: None needed.

Test Results: Symptoms are highly suggestive of osteoarthritis.

DIAGNOSIS: OSTEOARTHRITIS

Review Patient Location: The office is still the best location.

Order Treatments:

Acetaminophen therapy (oral and continuous)

Warm compresses

The case may cut off here or sooner. If it doesn't, continue with the following.

Secondary Orders: Use your list to recall that the patient is overweight and sedentary. Prescribe a walking program and a weight-loss diet for the patient.

Advance Clock/Follow-up Appointment: Schedule an appointment in one month. After that, you can use the "call/see me as needed" option for advancing the clock until the case ends.

CASE 7

Initial Presentation and Contributing History: A 65-year-old male comes to the emergency department with chest pain radiating to the jaw and shortness of breath.

Vital Signs:

Temp: 38°C (100.4°F)	BP systolic: 110 mmHg
Pulse: 89 beats/min; regular rhythm	BP diastolic: 86 mmHg
Respiratory rate: 26/min	Height: 178 cm (70 in)
	Weight: 72 kg (158 lbs)

The pain began four hours ago when the patient was cleaning his garage. The pain came on abruptly and is still present. The patient has a history of angina and hypertension. He takes nitroglycerin as needed and hydrochlorothiazide daily. His current pain doesn't respond to nitroglycerin. He smokes two packs per day. The rest of the history is noncontributory. *(Reminder: make your list now.)*

Patient Location: Chest pain can indicate a life-threatening condition, and the patient may benefit from immediate intervention. The emergency department is the best place for now.

Physical Exam: The patient may need immediate treatment, so perform a focused physical exam including general appearance, chest/lungs, heart/cardiovascular, and abdomen. Complete the exam later. On exam, he is diaphoretic and anxious. An S_4 heart sound is audible. The rest of the exam is normal.

Differential Diagnosis: Myocardial infarct, angina, pulmonary embolism, aortic dissection

CASE 7 (continued)

Order Tests:

Chest x-ray (CXR) (order as stat)

Cardiac enzymes, serum (order as stat every 8 hours × 3)

Electrocardiogram (ECG) (order as stat)

Basic metabolic profile (Chem 7) (order as stat)

Complete blood count (CBC) (order as stat)

Use the "call with next available result" option after you've ordered the tests, and begin treatment as soon as you know the diagnosis.

Test Results:

CXR: Mildly enlarged heart, no widened mediastinum, normal aortic arch

Impression: Mild cardiomegaly

Cardiac enzymes:

Creatine kinase, serum, total: 60 U/L (nl = 10–70)

Creatine kinase, myocardial band: 35 U/L (nl < 5% total)

ECG: Sinus tachycardia, regular rhythm, and ST elevation

Interpretation: Acute myocardial ischemia

Chem 7: Normal

CBC: Normal

DIAGNOSIS: ACUTE MYOCARDIAL INFARCTION

Review Patient Location: Treatment can begin in the emergency department, and the patient can be transferred to the ward when he is stable.

CASE 7 (continued)

Order Treatments:

IV access

Vital signs (order as stat every hour)

Oxygen (inhalation and continuous)

Nitroglycerin (NTG) (sublingual and continuous)

Morphine (IV and continuous)

Aspirin therapy (oral and continuous)

Heparin therapy (IV and continuous)

Metoprolol (IV and continuous)

Captopril (oral and continuous)

Consent for procedure

Cardiology consult

Angioplasty, balloon catheter (PTCA)

Monitor, cardiac (telemetry)

The case may cut off here or sooner. If it doesn't, continue with the following.

Secondary Orders: Use your list to recall that the patient smokes. Educate the patient about smoking cessation. He may also need a lipid profile (with treatment if necessary), low sodium/cholesterol diet, low-level activity, sexual abstinence, and laxatives.

Advance Clock/Follow-up Appointment: The patient can be discharged home after three to four days of continued improvement. Schedule the patient to return in 10 days for an exercise stress test before allowing him to return to normal activity. After that, you can use the "call/see me as needed" option for advancing the clock until the case ends.

CASE 8

Initial Presentation and Contributing History: A 70-year-old male with a history of congestive heart failure presents to the emergency department with worsening shortness of breath.

Vital Signs:

Temp: 37°C (98.6°F)	BP systolic: 140 mmHg
Pulse: 87 beats/min; regular rhythm	BP diastolic: 88 mmHg
Respiratory rate: 22/min	Height: 175 cm (69 in)
	Weight: 72 kg (158 lbs)

The patient has a long history of hypertension and coronary artery disease. He was diagnosed with heart failure two months ago when he began experiencing shortness of breath. He underwent extensive testing and is scheduled to see his doctor in one week. His condition had been stable until two days ago when he developed a dry cough. He now wakes up during the night short of breath, and has difficulty climbing stairs without resting. He has no other symptoms. He was prescribed metoprolol but admits to missing occasional doses. He takes no other medications. The rest of the history is noncontributory. *(Reminder: make your list now.)*

Patient Location: The emergency department is a suitable place for the patient until the severity of his condition is better characterized.

Physical Exam: The patient is stable so perform a complete physical exam. On exam the patient is sitting comfortably. His jugular veins are distended. A prominent S_3 heart sound is audible, and his cardiac apex is displaced laterally. There are dullness and rales in both lung bases. Both lower extremities are cool with mild pitting edema. The rest of the exam is normal.

CASE 8 (continued)

Differential Diagnosis: Heart failure exacerbation due to worsening heart failure, myocardial ischemia, valve disease, cardiomyopathy

Order Tests:

> Basic metabolic profile (Chem 7) (order as routine)
>
> Complete blood count (CBC) (order as routine)
>
> Chest x-ray (CXR) (order as routine)
>
> Electrocardiogram (ECG) (order as routine)

Use the "call with next available result" option after you've ordered the tests, and begin treatment as soon as you know the diagnosis.

Test Results:

> Chem 7: Urea nitrogen: 20.0 mg/dL (nl = 7–18), creatinine: 2.0 mg/dL (nl = 0.6–1.2), sodium: 136 mEq/L (nl = 136–145), potassium: 4.0 mEq/L (nl = 3.5–5.0)
>
> CBC: Normal
>
> CXR: Cardiomegaly, enlarged pulmonary vessels, bilateral pleural effusions
>
> Impression: Congestive heart failure
>
> ECG: Regular rhythm, normal QRS, nonspecific ST-T wave changes
>
> Interpretation: No acute ischemia

DIAGNOSIS: CONGESTIVE HEART FAILURE

Review Patient Location: The patient should be admitted to the ward for control of his symptoms.

CASE 8 (continued)

Order Treatments:

Oxygen (inhalation and continuous)

Captopril (oral and continuous)

Furosemide (oral and continuous)

Spironolactone (oral and continuous)

Hydralazine (oral and continuous)

Metoprolol (oral and continuous)

Low-salt diet

Weight (daily)

Basic metabolic profile (Chem 7) (every 12 hours)

Fluid restriction

Echocardiography (routine)

The case may cut off here or sooner. If it doesn't, continue with the following.

Secondary Orders: Use your list to recall that the patient was skipping medication doses. Counsel the patient about medication compliance.

Advance Clock/Follow-up Appointment: Send the patient home when his symptoms have improved. Schedule the patient to return in one week. After that, you can use the "call/see me as needed" option for advancing the clock until the case ends.

CASE 9

Initial Presentation and Contributing History: A 20-year-old female presents to your office with urinary frequency, urgency, and burning.

Vital Signs:

Temp: 37°C (98.6°F)	BP systolic: 118 mmHg
Pulse: 74 beats/min; regular rhythm	BP diastolic: 66 mmHg
Respiratory rate: 20/min	Height: 172 cm (68 in)
	Weight: 59 kg (130 lbs)

The patient, who is otherwise healthy, reports a gradual onset of symptoms beginning three days ago. She denies other symptoms including fever, chills, nausea, vomiting, flank pain, hematuria, or vaginal discharge. She is sexually active with multiple partners and denies any prior pregnancies, renal stones, sexually transmitted diseases, or urinary tract infections. She is taking no medication, and is allergic to sulfa drugs. The rest of the history is noncontributory. *(Reminder: make your list now.)*

Patient Location: This patient's condition is not emergent, therefore, she can remain in your office for a complete evaluation.

Physical Exam: The patient is stable, so perform a complete physical exam. On exam, she is not acutely distressed. Her abdomen is soft with mild suprapubic tenderness. She has no flank tenderness. The rest of the exam is normal.

Differential Diagnosis: Lower urinary tract infection, vaginitis, urethritis, pyelonephritis

CASE 9 (continued)

Order Tests:

> Complete blood count (CBC) (order as routine)
>
> Urinalysis (UA) (order as routine)
>
> Urine Gram stain (order as routine)
>
> Urine culture (order as routine)
>
> Basic metabolic profile (Chem 7) (order as routine)
>
> HCG, serum, qualitative (pregnancy test) (order as routine)

Use the "call with next available result" option after you've ordered the tests and begin treatment as soon as you know the diagnosis.

Test Results:

> CBC: White cell count 11000/mm^3 (nl = 3500–10500)
>
> UA: Acid pH, positive protein, leukocytes, and leukocyte esterase
>
> Urine Gram stain: Leukocytes and gram-negative rods
>
> Urine culture: Pending
>
> Chem 7: Normal
>
> Pregnancy test: Negative

DIAGNOSIS: LOWER URINARY TRACT INFECTION

Review Patient Location: Treatment can begin in your office; the patient can be sent home.

CASE 9 (continued)

Order Treatments:

Ciprofloxacin (oral and continuous)
Hydration (oral)

The case may cut off here or sooner. If it doesn't, continue with the following.

Secondary Orders: Use your list to recall that the patient has multiple sex partners. Counsel the patient about safe-sex practices.

Advance Clock/Follow-up Appointment: Advance the clock until the culture results are reported. After that, you can use the "call/see me as needed" option for advancing the clock until the case ends.

CASE 10

Initial Presentation and Contributing History: A 54-year-old male presents to the emergency department with dyspnea, fatigue, syncope, and black-colored emesis. He is restless and appears pale.

Vital Signs:

Temp: 37°C (98.6°F)	BP systolic: 104 mmHg
Pulse: 105 beats/min; regular rhythm	BP diastolic: 60 mmHg
Respiratory rate: 26/min	Height: 188 cm (74 in)
	Weight: 84 kg (185 lbs)

The patient's symptoms have been present for one day. He has a long history of alcohol use and has had similar episodes before. He also has osteoarthritis for which he takes ibuprofen. He smokes one pack of cigarettes per day. He denies prior liver disease and blood-clotting disorders. The rest of the history is noncontributory. *(Reminder: make your list now.)*

Patient Location: This patient's condition could be life threatening; he should, therefore, remain in the emergency department for a complete evaluation.

Physical Exam: Based on the patient's vital signs, he may need immediate intervention. Perform a focused physical exam including general appearance, chest/lungs, heart/cardiovascular, and abdomen. Complete the exam later. On exam, he is alert, diaphoretic, and pale. He is tachycardic, and has mild abdominal distension with epigastric tenderness. Rectal exam reveals no occult blood. The rest of the exam is normal.

Differential Diagnosis: Gastrointestinal bleeding due to peptic ulcer disease, esophageal varices, or Mallory-Weiss tears.

CASE 10 (continued)

Order Tests:

Orthostatic vitals (order as stat)
Basic metabolic profile (Chem 7) (order as routine)
Aspartate aminotransferase (AST) (order as routine)
Alanine aminotransferase (ALT) (order as routine)
Prothrombin time (PT) (order as stat)
Partial thromboplastin time (PTT) (order as stat)
Nasogastric tube with suction (order as stat)
Gastric lavage (order as stat)
Vital signs (every hour)
Complete blood count (CBC) (order as stat)
Blood type and crossmatch

Use the "call with next available result" option after you've ordered
the tests, and begin treatment as soon as you know the diagnosis.

Test Results:

Orthostatic vitals: Supine pulse 84 and BP 114/66; upright
pulse 105 and BP 102/62
Chem 7: Normal
AST: Normal
ALT: Normal
PT: Normal
PTT: Normal
Gastric lavage: Dark red and black semisolid material
CBC: Hemoglobin 6 gm/dl (nl = 13–17); hematocrit 19% (nl = 40–52)
Blood type: O+

CASE 10 (continued)

DIAGNOSIS: UPPER GASTROINTESTINAL BLEED

Review Patient Location: The patient needs frequent monitoring; he should be admitted to intensive care.

Order Treatments:

IV fluids (normal saline)

Transfuse packed red blood cells

NPO

Consent for procedure

Gastroenterology consult

Upper gastrointestinal endoscopy

Omeprazole (oral and continuous)

Discontinue ibuprofen

The case may cut off here or sooner. If it doesn't, continue with the following.

Secondary Orders: Use your list to recall that the patient smokes and uses alcohol. Counsel the patient about limiting alcohol use and smoking cessation.

Advance Clock/Follow-up Appointment: Follow the patient's vital signs and hemoglobin/hematocrit levels until he is hemodynamically stable. Transfer the patient to the hospital ward. After that, you can use the "call/see me as needed" option for advancing the clock until the case ends.

CASE 11

Initial Presentation and Contributing History: A 25-year-old female presents to the emergency department with a 12-hour history of right lower quadrant abdominal pain, nausea, and vomiting. The pain was initially localized to the mid abdomen. She is lying supine and says it hurts to move.

Vital Signs:

Temp: 38.7°C (101.6°F)	BP systolic: 130 mmHg
Pulse: 90 beats/min; regular rhythm	BP diastolic: 86 mmHg
Respiratory rate: 20/min	Height: 168 cm (66 in)
	Weight: 95 kg (210 lbs)

The patient, who is otherwise healthy, first noticed the symptoms about 12 hours ago during lunch. She has not eaten since. She has never had similar symptoms before. Her last bowel movement was yesterday and it was normal. She has never had surgery before. She is sexually active with one partner and uses condoms regularly for birth control. The rest of the history is noncontributory. *(Reminder: make your list now.)*

Patient Location: The emergency department is the best place until the patient's condition has been fully evaluated.

Physical Exam: The patient is in severe pain, so perform a focused physical exam including general appearance, chest/lungs, heart/cardiovascular, abdomen, and genitalia. Complete the exam later. On exam, she is overweight, pale, alert, and lying still. There is right lower quadrant abdominal pain diffusely with palpation and rebound tenderness. No masses are detected. The patient offers significant muscular resistance to palpation. The rest of the exam is normal.

CASE 11 (continued)

Differential Diagnosis: Acute appendicitis, gastroenteritis, pyelonephritis, nephrolithiasis, pelvic inflammatory disease, ovarian cyst, ectopic pregnancy

Order Tests:

> Complete blood count (CBC) (order as routine)
>
> Basic metabolic profile (Chem 7) (order as routine)
>
> Urinalysis (UA) (order as routine)
>
> HCG, serum, qualitative (pregnancy test) (order as stat)
>
> Computed tomography, abdomen (CT scan) (order as stat)

Use the "call with next available result" option after you've ordered the tests, and begin treatment as soon as you know the diagnosis.

Test Results:

> CBC: White count 12000 mm^3 (nl − 3500–10500)
>
> Chem 7: Normal
>
> UA: Normal
>
> Pregnancy test: Negative
>
> Abdominal CT scan: Enlarged appendix with wall enhancement and surrounding inflammation
>
> Impression: Acute appendicitis

DIAGNOSIS: ACUTE APPENDICITIS

Review Patient Location: The patient needs surgical intervention. Transfer the patient to the hospital ward after surgery.

CASE 11 (continued)

Order Treatments:

IV fluids (normal saline)

Morphine (IV and continuous)

Cefazolin (IV and continuous)

NPO

Consent for procedure

General surgery consult

Laproscopic appendectomy

The case may cut off here or sooner. If it doesn't, continue with the following.

Secondary Orders: Use your list to recall that the patient is overweight. Counsel the patient about diet and exercise.

Advance Clock/Follow-up Appointment: Keep the patient in the hospital until she has recovered from surgery. Schedule follow-up appointment 10 days after discharge. After that, you can use the "call/see me as needed" option for advancing the clock until the case ends.

CASE 12

Initial Presentation and Contributing History: A 66-year-old female is brought to the emergency department by her husband because she is confused and can't move her left leg or arm.

Vital Signs:

Temp: 38°C (100.4°F)	BP systolic: 154 mmHg
Pulse: 85 beats/min; regular rhythm	BP diastolic: 94 mmHg
Respiratory rate: 22/min	Height: 168 cm (66 in)
	Weight: 93 kg (205 lbs)

The patient's husband says her symptoms started three hours ago. Her leg was involved first, and the symptoms appear to be progressing. The patient seems unaware that there is anything wrong. The patient smokes cigarettes and has a history of hypertension, atherosclerosis, and one myocardial infarct that occurred years ago. The patient denies recent trauma. The rest of the history is noncontributory. *(Reminder: make your list now.)*

Patient Location: The emergency department is the best place until the patient's condition has been fully evaluated.

Physical Exam: The patient's condition is evolving, so perform a focused physical exam including general appearance, chest/lungs, heart/cardiovascular, and neuro/psych. Complete the exam later. On exam, she is overweight, alert, and confused about where she is. Carotid bruits are present bilaterally. Her strength and sensation are significantly reduced in the left leg and moderately reduced in the left arm. Her right arm and leg are unaffected. The rest of the exam is normal.

Differential Diagnosis: Transient ischemic attack, cerebral infarct, intracranial hemorrhage

CASE 12 (continued)

Order Tests:

> Complete blood count (CBC) (order as routine)
>
> Basic metabolic profile (Chem 7) (order as routine)
>
> Prothrombin time (PT) (order as stat)
>
> Partial thromboplastin time (PTT) (order as stat)
>
> Electrocardiogram (ECG) (order as stat)
>
> Computed tomography, head (CT scan) (order as stat)
>
> Doppler, carotid arteries (order as stat)

Use the "call with next available result" option after you've ordered the tests, and begin treatment as soon as you know the diagnosis.

Test Results:

> CBC: Normal
>
> Chem 7: Normal
>
> PT: Normal
>
> PTT: Normal
>
> ECG: Regular rhythm, isolated Q waves, normal QRS complexes, normal ST waves
>
> Interpretation: Old myocardial infarct; no acute ischemia
>
> Head CT scan: Old right-sided cerebral infarct, no acute infarct, hemorrhage, infection, aneurysm, or mass
>
> Impression: No acute changes
>
> Carotid Doppler: Significantly reduced flow velocity in both carotid arteries

DIAGNOSIS: CEREBRAL ISCHEMIA

Review Patient Location: The patient should be admitted to the hospital ward for treatment.

CASE 12 (continued)

Order Treatments:

Oxygen (inhalation and continuous)

Pulse oximetry

IV fluids (normal saline)

Aspirin

NPO

Cefazolin (IV and continuous)

Vascular surgery consult

Consent for procedure

Thromboendarterectomy, carotid (routine)

The case may cut off here or sooner. If it doesn't, continue with the following:

Secondary Orders: Use your list to recall that the patient is overweight and smokes. Counsel about diet, exercise, and smoking cessation.

Advance Clock/Follow-up Appointment: Keep the patient in the hospital until she has recovered from surgery. Schedule a follow-up appointment one week after discharge. After that, you can use the "call/see me as needed" option for advancing the clock until the case ends.

CASE 13

Initial Presentation and Contributing History: A 4-month-old male is brought to the emergency room by his mother for a gradual onset of fever, irritability, lethargy, and difficulty feeding.

Vital Signs:

Temp: 40°C (104.0°F)	BP systolic: 92 mmHg
Pulse: 92 beats/min; regular rhythm	BP diastolic: 60 mmHg
Respiratory rate: 22/min	Height: 64 cm (25 in)
	Weight: 7 kg (15 lbs)

The symptoms began three days ago and seem to be getting worse. The child has been healthy except for an ear infection that started 10 days ago. The family pediatrician prescribed a liquid medication to treat the ear infection. The mother reports giving the child a few doses and then stopping after the child seemed to get better. The patient has two brothers who attend day care. The mother reports a normal pregnancy and delivery. The patient is up to date on all vaccinations, and there is no history of head trauma. The rest of the history is noncontributory. *(Reminder: make your list now.)*

Patient Location: The patient's problem is not yet well defined. The emergency department is the best place until his condition is better characterized.

Physical Exam: The patient is stable, so do a complete physical exam. On exam the patient is well developed, hypotonic, crying, and appears ill. His left tympanic membrane is erythematous and bulging with a diminished light reflex. His fontanelle is bulging, and his neck is stiff. The rest of the exam is normal.

CASE 13 (continued)

Differential Diagnosis: Otitis media and meningitis, CNS mass lesion (abscess, tumor, or hematoma), intoxication

Order Tests:

Complete blood count (CBC) (order as routine)

Basic metabolic profile (Chem 7) (order as routine)

Lumbar puncture (order as stat)

CSF Gram stain (order as stat)

CSF protein (order as stat)

CSF glucose (order as stat)

CSF cell count (order as stat)

CSF culture, bacterial (order as routine)

CSF culture, fungal (order as routine)

Blood culture (order as routine)

Use the "call with next available result" option after you've ordered the tests, and begin treatment as soon as you have enough information to do so.

Test Results:

CBC: White cell count $19000/mm^3$ (nl = 3500–10500)

Chem 7: Normal

Lumbar puncture: Opening pressure 240 mm water; 3 mL of turbid fluid obtained

CSF Gram stain: Gram-positive diplococci

CSF protein: 150 mg/dL (nl = 0–40)

CSF glucose: 32 mg/dL (nl = 40–70)

CSF cell count: $>500/mm^3$ (nl < 3)

CSF culture results: Pending

Blood culture results: Pending

CASE 13 (continued)

DIAGNOSIS: BACTERIAL MENINGITIS

Review Patient Location: This patient has a potentially life-threatening infection, and should be admitted to the hospital ward for treatment.

Order Treatments:

IV fluids (1/4 normal saline)

Dexamethasone (IV and continuous)

Ceftriaxone (IV and continuous)

Vancomycin (IV and continuous)

Tylenol (oral and continuous)

The case may cut off here or sooner. If it doesn't, continue with the following.

Secondary Orders: Use your list to recall that the mother stopped the child's treatment for his ear infection before it was finished. Educate the mother about medication compliance.

Advance Clock/Follow-up Appointment: Monitor the patient until his symptoms have improved and his fever is gone. Discharge the patient. After that, you can use the "call/see me as needed" option for advancing the clock until the case ends.

CASE 14

Initial Presentation and Contributing History: A 37-year-old male comes to the emergency department with severe abdominal pain.

Vital Signs:

Temp: 37.5°C (99.5°F)	BP systolic: 106 mmHg
Pulse: 86 beats/min; regular rhythm	BP diastolic: 84 mmHg
Respiratory rate: 20/min	Height: 178 cm (70 in)
	Weight: 54 kg (120 lbs)

The pain is in his epigastrium and began three days ago. It is a dull, continuous pain and radiates to his lower back. He feels nauseated, and he has had two episodes of vomiting. The patient drinks five glasses of bourbon each day and first noticed the pain after a particularly heavy night of drinking. He is otherwise healthy and takes no medications. He denies hematemesis or melena. The rest of the history is noncontributory. *(Reminder: make your list now.)*

Patient Location: The patient's problem is not yet well defined. The emergency department is the best place until his condition is better characterized.

Physical Exam: The patient is stable, so do a complete physical exam. On exam he is thin, cachectic, and in obvious pain. There is dullness to percussion over the left lower hemithorax. His abdomen is flat and markedly tender over the epigastrium. No abdominal masses are palpated. Bowel sounds are diminished. Rectal exam is negative for occult blood. The rest of the exam is normal.

Differential Diagnosis: Alcoholic pancreatitis, cholecytitis, gastritis, peptic ulcer disease

CASE 14 (continued)

Order Tests:

> Complete blood count (CBC) (order as routine)
>
> Basic metabolic profile (Chem 7) (order as routine)
>
> Calcium (order as routine)
>
> Magnesium (order as routine)
>
> Amylase, serum (order as routine)
>
> Lipase, serum (order as routine)
>
> Aspartate aminotransferase (AST) (order as routine)
>
> Alanine aminotransferase (ALT) (order as routine)
>
> Alkaline phosphatase, serum (order as routine)
>
> Bilirubin, serum, total and direct (order as routine)
>
> Computed tomography, abdomen (CT scan) (order as routine)
>
> Blood gasses, arterial (order as routine)

Use the "call with next available result" option after you've ordered the tests, and begin treatment as soon as you have enough information to do so.

Test Results:

> CBC: White cell count 14000/mm^3 (nl = 3500–10500)
>
> Chem 7: Glucose 180 mg/dL (nl = 70–110)
>
> Calcium: 8.0 mg/dL (nl = 8.4–10.2)
>
> Magnesium: 0.9 mEq/L (nl = 1.5–2.0)
>
> Amylase, serum: 670 U/L (nl = 30–110)
>
> Lipase, serum: 830 U/L (nl = 5–208)
>
> Aspartate aminotransferase (AST): 216 U/L (nl = 15.0–40.0)
>
> Alanine aminotransferase (ALT): 110 U/L (nl = 10.0–40.0)
>
> Alkaline phosphatase, serum: 225 U/L (nl = 20–115)
>
> Bilirubin, serum, total and direct: Total: 3.0 mg/dL (nl = 0.1–1.0); direct: 1.1mg/dL (nl = 0.0–0.3)

CASE 14 (continued)

CT scan, abdomen: Diffuse pancreatic enlargement with focal irregularities and a small peripancreatic fluid collection. The gallbladder and ducts are free of stones. Mild left pleural effusion with atelectasis. Normal sized liver, spleen, and kidneys with no defects. No masses or calcifications are present.

Impression: Acute pancreatitis with focal necrosis and edema

Arterial blood gasses: Normal

DIAGNOSIS: ACUTE PANCREATITIS

Review Patient Location: The patient should be admitted to the hospital ward.

Order Treatments:

IV normal saline

NPO

Nasogastric suction

Ranitidine (IV and continuous)

Meperidine (IV and continuous)

Calcium chloride (IV and continuous)

Magnesium supplement (IV and continuous)

Promethazine hydrochloride (IV and continuous)

The case may cut off here or sooner. If it doesn't, continue with the following.

Secondary Orders: Use your list to recall that the patient is cachectic and uses alcohol heavily. Order alcohol abstinence and a multivitamin. Educate the patient about alcohol abuse and a proper diet.

Advance Clock/Follow-up Appointment: See the patient frequently to monitor symptoms, blood gasses, and other labs until his symptoms are gone. After that, you can use the "call/see me as needed" option for advancing the clock until the case ends.

CASE 15

Initial Presentation and Contributing History: A 24-year-old female comes to your office complaining of hot flashes and missed menses.

Vital Signs:

Temp: 38°C (100.4°F)	BP systolic: 142 mmHg
Pulse: 82 beats/min; irregular rhythm	BP diastolic: 86 mmHg
Respiratory rate: 20/min	Height: 165 cm (65 in)
	Weight: 54 kg (118 lbs)

The hot flashes began about six months ago and seem to be getting more frequent. She previously had regular menstrual periods. She first had bouts of irregular menstrual bleeding and has missed her period for the past two months. She has become increasingly restless and anxious with occasional chest discomfort and palpitations. She also reports an unintentional 10-pound (4.5 kg) weight loss. The patient is a graduate student and drinks one pot of coffee per day to stay awake. She has never been pregnant. She is sexually active with one partner and takes an oral contraceptive. The rest of the history is noncontributory. *(Reminder: make your list now.)*

Patient Location: The patient is stable and needs further testing. She should remain in your office.

Physical Exam: The patient is stable, so do a complete physical exam. On exam she is thin, mildly diaphoretic, and sitting comfortably. She has proptosis of the eyes and eyelid retraction bilaterally. A diffusely enlarged, nontender thyroid gland is noted. Loud S_1 and S_2 heart sounds are heard. There is a mid systolic murmur and a sporadically occurring extra heart sound. She has a fine tremor in her fingers and brisk tendon reflexes. Mild nonpitting edema is present in her lower extremities. The rest of the exam is normal.

CASE 15 (continued)

Differential Diagnosis: Hyperthyroidism (Graves' disease, multi-nodular goiter, thyroid adenoma, thyroiditis), pregnancy

Order Tests:

Basic metabolic profile (Chem 7) (order as routine)

Thyroid stimulating hormone, serum (TSH) (order as routine)

Thyroxine, serum, free (free T_4) (order as routine)

Electrocardiogram (ECG) (order as routine)

Pregnancy test (order as routine)

Radioactive iodine uptake (order as routine)

Use the "call with next available result" option after you've ordered the tests, and begin treatment as soon as you have enough information to do so.

Test Results:

Chem 7: Normal

TSH: 0.03 μU/L (nl = 0.5–5.0)

Free T_4: 3.7 ng/dL (nl = 0.8–2.4)

ECG: Irregular rhythm, early abnormal P waves, normal QRS complexes, normal ST waves

Impression: Premature atrial contractions

Pregnancy test: Negative

Thyroid uptake: 53%/24 hr (nl = 5–30)

DIAGNOSIS: GRAVES' HYPERTHYROIDISM

Review Patient Location: This patient should be treated as an outpatient.

CASE 15 (continued)

Order Treatments:

> Propranolol (oral and continuous)
> Radioactive iodine (^{131}I) (oral and once)

The case may cut off here or sooner. If it doesn't, continue with the following.

Secondary Orders: Use your list to recall that the patient drinks one pot of coffee per day. Counsel the patient about limiting her caffeine intake.

Advance Clock/Follow-up Appointment: Schedule the patient to return at six-week intervals for reassessment of symptoms, TSH, and free T$_4$. After that, you can use the "call/see me as needed" option for advancing the clock until the case ends.

Appendix: Review Resources

Most board review books consist of factual information presented either in brief bulleted lists or text descriptions of diseases by subject. Information presented in either format is a great way to review for multiple-choice questions and expand your fund of knowledge for case-based testing. Once you know the facts, case presentations that closely mimic the CCS may be a more beneficial review format. The very best source of practice cases for the CCS is the one provided by the examiners online or on the practice CD you receive when you apply for the exam. The examiners provide only a few cases, but they are excellent for practicing with the exam format (making orders, getting test results, etc.). After you have worked each case once or twice you will begin to memorize the patients' diseases and responses and further review of those cases is of little benefit. The practice cases in this book are designed to provide you with more case-based material in a format that is similar to the CCS. Additionally, there are several Internet sites that offer case presentations of common medical problems in a step-by-step format. Box A.1 lists Internet sites with cases that you may find helpful for your CCS review.

BOX A.1	ONLINE CCS REVIEW SOURCES
http://www.familypractice.com
http://info.med.yale.edu/intmed/education/casebooks.html
http://www.people.virginia.edu/~smb4v/casemenu.html
http://www.kcom.edu/faculty/chamberlain/cases.htm

The way the cases are presented at each site varies, and some are better approximations of the CCS than others. Additionally, numerous books that aren't specifically board review books provide case-based reviews. There should be no shortage of case-based material for you to use for your review. Use the cases the examiners provide to familiarize yourself with the test format, and then explore other books and Internet sources for more cases.

References

1. USMLE. Federation of State Medical Boards of the United States and National Board of Medical Examiners. Available at: http://www.usmle.org. Accessed April 15, 2003.

2. O'Donnell MJ, Obenshain SS, Erdmann JB. Background essential to the proper use of results of step 1 and step 2 of the USMLE. Acad Med 1993;68:734–749.

3. Clyman SG, Melnick DE, Clauser BE. Computer-based case simulations from medicine: Assessing skills in patient management. In: Tekian A, McGuire CH, McGahie WC, eds. Innovative Simulations for Assessing Professional Competence. Chicago: University of Illinois, Department of Medical Education, 1999:29–41.

4. Clyman SG, Melnick DE, Clauser BE. Computer-based case simulations. In: Mancall, EL. Assessing Clinical Reasoning: The Oral Examination and Alternative Methods. Evanston: American Board of Medical Specialties, 1995:139–149.

5. Clauser BE, Margolis MJ, Swanson DB. An examination of the contribution of computer-based case simulations to the USMLE step 3 examination. Acad Med 2002;77(suppl): S80–82.

6. Wainer H, Thissen D. Combining multiple-choice and constructed-response test scores: toward a Marxist theory of test construction. Appl Meas Educ 1993;6:103–118.

Index

Index note: Page references with a b indicate a box on designated page.

Acute appendicitis, sample case of, 58–60

Acute myocardial infarction, sample case of, 46–48

Acute pancreatitis, sample case of, 67–70

Advancing the clock during a timed test, 15–16

Asthma, sample case of, 41–43

Bacterial meningitis, sample case of, 64–66

Cancer, as realistic exam topic, 27

Case ending
implications of, 16–17, 27–28
as part of timed test, 7, 12, 28
taking notes for secondary problems, 6b, 7

Cases
anticipating and predicting case topics of, 26–27
implications of abrupt/cut-off ending of, 16–17, 27–28
initial management phase of, 5–6, 6b, 7–13
practice sample cases for, 27–72
watching and waiting phase, 12–13, 15–17

Cerebral ischemia, sample case of, 61–63

Community-acquired pneumonia, sample case of, 29–31

Computer-Based Case Simulation (CCS)
online practice cases for, 73b, xii
scoring of, 24, 24b, 25
two-stage approach to conquering CCS, 5–6, 6b, 7–13

Congestive heart failure, sample case of, 48–51

Consults, ordering of, 10–11

Daily visits, scheduling of, 15

Diabetic ketoacidosis, sample case of, 35–37

Differential diagnosis
formulating during initial management stage, 6b, 8–9
See also specific sample cases

Drugs/medications, ordering during treatment, 11

Exam, preparing for
effects of clinical training as preparation for, 1, 2
for international medical graduates (IMGs), 3–4
post medical school training for, 1
practicing with sample tests, 18–20, 20b, 21, 26–72
pre-exam requirements for, 1–2
"Rule of Twos" of studying for, 2
selecting a state medical board for, 2

Fluids, ordering during
   treatment, 11
Follow-up appointments,
   scheduling of, 13–14, 16–17

Gastrointestinal bleed, upper,
   sample case of, 55–57
Graves hyperthyroidism, sample
   case of, 70–72

Health maintenance, assessing
   for, 13
Hyperthyroidism, sample
   case of, 70–72

Initial management stage
   reading the introductory
      statement and patient
      history, 5–6, 6b
   taking notes during, 6, 6b, 7
   determine setting/location for
      treatment, 6b, 7–8
   performing the physical
      exam, 6b, 8
   formulating a differential
      diagnosis, 6b, 8–9
   ordering tests, 6b, 9–10
   reevaluate setting/location
      of treatment, 10
   ordering treatment, 6b,
      10–12
International medical graduates
   (IMGs), preparation for CCS
   examination for, 3–4

Laboratory values, interpretation
   and reporting of, 9
Location/setting of treatment
   initial determination of, 6b, 7–8
   reevaluating again, 10
Lower urinary tract infection,
   sample case of, 52–54

Managing time
   in completing a case, 16–17
   implication of abrupt ending
      of cases, 7, 12, 28
   techniques in advancing the
      clock, 15–16
Meningitis, bacterial, sample case
   of, 64–66
Myocardial infarction, acute,
   sample case of, 46–48

Note taking
   in addressing secondary
      problems, 12–13
   during initial management
      stage, 6, 6b, 7

Obstetric consults, 11
Orders/ordering
   managing CCS test aspects
      of, 18–20, 20b, 21
   practicing with sample cases, 19
   recognized by the CCS, 20b
Osteoarthritis, sample
   case of, 44–45

Pancreatitis, acute, sample case
   of, 67–70
Patient complaints
   in CCS patient cases, 5–6, 6b
   See also specific sample cases
Patient counseling, ordering
   of, 13
Patient education, ordering
   of, 13
Patient history
   in CCS patient cases, 5–6, 6b
   See also specific sample cases
Physical exam
   during initial management
      stage, 6b, 8
   reexamination of patient with,

Pneumonia, community-acquired, sample case of, 29–31

Practice and sample cases
approximating CCS reality with, 19
cut-off point in sample cases, 27–28
experimenting with, 19
how to read and process, 28
order lists generated in CCS, 20–21
sample cases for, 27–72

Psychiatric illness, as realistic exam topic, 27

Reality versus CCS
approximating reality of the test, 19
details overlooked, 18–20, 20b, 21
familiarizing with CCS software, 19
managing CCS test aspects when writing orders, 18–20, 20b, 21
orders lists in CCS, 20b

Real time, 14

Ruptured ectopic pregnancy, sample case of, 32–34

Sample practice. See Practice and samples

Scheduling, reevaluating patients during watching and waiting stage, 15–16

Scoring
CCS scoring key of, 24, 24b, 25
determination of passing scores in, 23
of multiple-choice questions, 22–23, 23b
pilot-tested questions in, 23

scores for each case in, 24
USMLE reported as a scaled score, 22

Secondary problems
managing during watching and waiting stage, 12–13
taking notes in initial management stage, 6, 6b, 7

Setting/location of treatment
initial determination of, 6b, 7–8
reevaluating again, 10

Splenic rupture, sample case of, 38–40

Surgery, ordering consult during treatment, 11

Taking notes
addressing secondary problems with, 12–13
during initial management stage, 5–6, 6b

Tests, ordering of
interpretation provided in the CCS test, 9
ordering during initial management stage, 6b, 9–10
scheduling reevaluation of, 15

Timed test
advancing the clock in, 15–16
case endings in, 7, 12, 28
managing time of, 14–17
real time, 14
simulated time of the test, 14
using notes of secondary problems, 6b, 7

Treatment
determining setting/location of, 6b, 7–8
ordering in the initial management stage, 10–12
reevaluating again, 10

United States Medical Licensing
  Examination (USMLE)
  CCS practice cases from, xii
  CCS preparation for
    international medical
    graduates (IMGs) with, 3–4
  final test score of, 25
  pre-CCS requirements of, 1
  reported as a scaled score, 22
Upper gastrointestinal bleed,
  sample case of, 55–57

Urinary tract infection, lower,
  sample case of, 52–54

Watching and waiting stage
  addressing secondary
    problems, 12–13
  advancing the clock
    during, 13
  completing a case, 16–17
  scheduling follow-up
    appointments, 13